HABITUAL STRENGTH

TIM ANDERSON

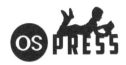

CONTENTS

DISCLAIMER!

You must get your physician's approval before beginning this exercise program.

These recommendations are not medical guidelines but are for educational purposes only. You must consult your physician prior to starting this program or if you have any medical condition or injury that is contraindicated to performing physical activity. This program is designed for healthy individuals eighteen years and older only.

See your physician before starting any exercise or nutrition program. If you are taking any medications, you must talk to your physician before starting any exercise program, including the *Habitual Strength* program. If you experience any lightheadedness, dizziness, or shortness of breath while exercising, stop the movement and consult a physician.

It is strongly recommended that you have a complete physical examination if you live a sedentary lifestyle, have high cholesterol, high blood pressure, diabetes, are overweight, or if you are over thirty years old. Please discuss all nutritional changes with your physician or a registered dietician. If your physician recommends that you not use the *Habitual Strength* program, please follow your doctor's orders.

All forms of exercise pose some inherent risks. The authors, editors, and publishers advise readers to take full responsibility for their own safety and know their limits. When using the exercises in this program, do not take risks beyond your level of experience, aptitude, training, and fitness. The exercises and dietary programs in this program are not intended as a substitute for any exercise routine, treatment, or dietary regimen prescribed by your physician.

FOREWORD BY DAN JOHN

I have known Tim Anderson for the better part of this past decade. We were teammates at a health and fitness certification, and we seemed to understand some basic things about the world of coaching and teaching. Firstly, that less is more, and, secondly, that if you can't explain what you have to offer to a six-year-old, you probably don't really understand the concept yourself.

I've enjoyed watching Tim's work evolve. When he first explained "pressing reset" to me, I did what you'll likely do, which is say "Isn't that great..." and promptly ignored him. Then my hip became necrotic and I faced a total hip replacement, and Tim became one of my go-to people. It's not a gentle procedure. The tools for this operation are found in hardware stores and the methods are so brutal you would be wise not have eaten before you watch the videos on it.

Following the surgery, I began following the Pressing RESET protocol. As soon as I could manage, I began breathing, rocking, and nodding. Every day, I got on the ground and did what I could. Every day. My doctor and therapist were amazed. My progress was astounding and when I showed them the moves, the reaction was interesting: "That's pretty good."

Pretty good? I can take pretty good. The fact that no other patient was progressing as quickly might have been a clue, but I'm not a medical doctor. I quickly lost the walker, the crutches, and the cane. During each and every workout, I was doing the

Resets. It took a while to get to march in place or skipping, but I was getting better every day.

One year later, I won the state Olympic lifting title. People with titanium hips are not supposed to get back on the medal stand much less the platform.

Habitual Strength is the next logical step in Tim's journey. You get all the insights of his continuing work, but you also get habits and nutritional insights plus ways to deal with your community.

The genius of the book is the programming. Tim maps out a reasonable, "do this" program that will put you back together. He has some rule-less rules about nutrition, and he lays out an outstanding program for resetting the body. Let me say this as simply as I can: this works. I am the proof. Moreover, you get some very interesting quotes in each chapter from *Star Trek* to *Matrix* to *Pirates of the Caribbean.*

Yes, it's simple. Yes, you've seen some of it before in other resources (often mine!) and, no, this isn't how Mr. Universe trains. But, outside of professional bodybuilding, the rest of us need this book.

Athletes can deal with travel issues, overtraining, and recovery problems by walking through the simple drills in this book. The elderly (Wait! That's me!) will get a new sense of movement and the tools for building a new body. Everybody else will get a vision of how simple, daily movements can add up to a better, healthier life.

Tim is a leader in fitness. Tim is a leader in the movement industry. Tim has chosen a path that isn't very sexy. It's solid and true. I can't think of a better voice in fitness to lead us back to the basics.

—Daniel John, Fulbright scholar and author of *Mass Made Simple, Easy Strength,* and *Never Let Go*

1

THE HABITS OF STRENGTH

...just as my strength was then, so now is my strength for war, both for going out and for coming in.

—Joshua 14:11

Every person was created to be strong and be in good health. We are all designed to develop, maintain, increase, and renew our strength through movement. *All movement is worthwhile, but each of us should focus on habitual movement. It is our daily habits, the movement routines we have that yield the level of strength and health we have.*

As a child, you once moved your way into a solid foundation of strength and resilience. Day in and day out, hour by hour, moment by moment, you learned how to move your way into being able to stand, walk, climb, and run. You moved to become strong, the stronger you became, the more you could move. The more you could move, the more strength you were able to develop. It was a wonderful cycle of habitual movement and resultant strength. You stopped moving only when you were resting and needing to recover, which also helped to further develop your strength.

As an adult, many of us no longer move to become strong. Many of us don't even move to maintain the strength we moved so much to gain in the beginning of our lives. The problem is, we are designed to move, and movement is what creates our health, vigor, and vitality—our strength. Yes, some people exercise to build strength, but exercise is a Band-Aid solution to a much bigger problem. When people lack strength, it's due to their developing habits that have removed their strength. Yes, exercise can make a person stronger, but it is almost a false type of strength, if it is not built on a foundation of habitual movement.

Can one hour of strength-training really overcome twenty-three hours of being sedentary? No, not really. Strength can be made, but it's not optimal strength and it will certainly be lacking in the complete picture of strength.

Having said that, it may be a good idea to offer what I mean by the word "strength." Strength is the ability to live life the way that you want to live it; to be able to move, think, work, play, love, and laugh throughout your entire life, regardless of your age.

My definition of strength is extremely hard to quantify. In fact, only one person is qualified to quantify it: you. Ultimately, you are the one who determines whether or not you are strong enough to live the way you want to live. No one else should be the judge of your own personal strength; no one else can live the life you want to live.

Ponder my definition of strength for a moment. Are you as strong and healthy as you want to be? Will your body allow you to live your life with the freedom that you want to enjoy? If not, this book is for you.

This is a book about reclaiming your strength, your health, through making easy neurological connections in your brain. You might call these connections "habits." The goal of this book is to help you learn how to establish ridiculously simple habits so you can restore your body's health and vigor—the strength you were born to have.

Also, throughout this book, the words "strength" and "health" will be used interchangeably. In my mind, they are the same thing. You cannot be healthy if you don't have strength, and you cannot have strength if you do not have health. So, for the purpose of this book, keep in mind that strength is more than a physical description of how much weight you can move. Strength is a description of the state and quality of your health. When a man feels "his strength return," he's really feeling his "health return," and vice versa.

Are you ready to feel your strength return? If so, it is time to remember the habits of strength and health.

2

HEALTH, HABITS, AND THE FREEDOM OF MOVEMENT

What strength do I have, that I should hope?

—Job 6:11

When the Dalai Lama answered the question about what surprises him most about humanity, he offered, "Man. Because he sacrifices his health in order to make money. Then he sacrifices money to recuperate his health. And then he is so anxious about the future that he does not enjoy the present; the result being that he does not live in the present or the future; he lives as if he is never going to die, and then he dies having never really lived."

This is a powerful statement. It highlights the value of life and good health, a value that money cannot rival. Money cannot buy happiness, or even contentment. Money cannot really even offer the joy of life's experiences. Only good health can.

If you have good health, you are free to focus on the things that matter in life. You can focus on your family, your community, and your job. If you don't have good health, all you can think about is how you want to be healthy. Poor health limits you from living life.

For example, have you ever been injured? Were you able to go about your normal life, as if nothing was wrong? Or did you focus on your injury throughout most of your days? It's not that you want to focus on an injury, but injuries and issues, when you have them, can invade all of your thoughts. Your thoughts become hijacked—and you begin to get really good at thinking these hijacked thoughts. There is a neurological reason for this, but we will discuss that later.

If you have never been injured, have you ever been sick? When you were sick, how loving and giving towards others were you? It is very hard to express love, gratitude, and selflessness when you're not feeling well. I'm not saying it's impossible to be loving and giving if your health is poor, but I am saying it is a whole lot easier to offer yourself to others when you have good health.

Many moons ago, I was a firefighter. We'd routinely answer EMS calls at local nursing homes. One of the most sobering things in the world is to see sixty-year-olds who are bedridden. Sixty isn't old! Sixty is the new fifty, and it should be like being forty. I often wondered what led people to end up unable to care for themselves. Yes, I know there're often extenuating circumstances that lead people to such places. I also know some people need care at relatively young ages because they've developed habits that have eroded their health and their freedom.

On the flipside of that coin is Jack LaLanne. Jack died in 2011 at the ripe, young age of ninety-six. You read that right. Jack was a young man when he passed away. Every single day of Jack's life was filled with the habits of strength. Jack moved like he was created to move. Even In his nineties, Jack could still perform fingertip pushups with his arms spread out like Superman. I would venture a guess that 97 percent of all twenty-year-olds in the world can't do that!

Jack never had to worry about living in a rest home because he always took care of himself. Every day, he practiced healthy habits. These habits led him to have a great quality of life well into his nineties. Jack didn't die because he was old. Jack died from pneumonia, and pneumonia doesn't discriminate between old and young. It's said the day before Jack died, he performed his daily workout routine.

Having good health enables you to live your life the way you want to live it. It allows you to play in the park with your kids. It allows you to love your spouse better, to be more neighborly, to be more productive—and it allows the freedom to stay out of a nursing home. Having good health allows you to live.

You were created to have good health, and you deserve to have good health. It is your responsibility to have and maintain your strength. You owe it to yourself, your family, your friends, and your community. In fact, your state of health influences and affects—or in some cases infects—the world around you, because your life is integrated with everyone you come into contact with.

Because you were made to be strong, you can improve your health regardless of your current health situation. It's easier than you think. You just need to know how to establish good, simple habits and make them stick. It's all about routine. We are a collection of what we do every day.

Years ago, I used to have a habit of eating fast-food burgers and ice cream several times a week. I worked out an hour a day, so I thought I could eat whatever I wanted. One day my wife walked by me, pinched my waist, and said, "Isn't that cute? You've got love handles!" I didn't care for that very much at all. My poor eating habit was accumulatively greater than my exercise habit. So, I made a change. I made a decision that day to change my eating habits, and I never looked back. Within months, I lost thirty pounds and, though I have never looked, I've never found the weight I lost.

My habits changed instantly. I am fortunate that I can flip a habit switch, at least in some areas. Not everyone can draw a hardline in the sand and instantly change their usual day-to-day routine. However, everyone is capable of changing his or her habits with continual, simple efforts. This is how you turn a mountain into a molehill: a shovelful of dirt and one rock at a time ...

You can build maintainable thought and movement habits that will serve you a lifetime. The first step to overcome mental inertia and make a habit stick is to resolve to change. Without that resolution—that initial desire—change is impossible, but once you resolve to change, you cannot fail to restore your health and vitality.

This takes patience. This takes "big picture" thinking. We'll first focus on small changes. These small changes serve as the catalyst for larger changes later on. Becoming healthy and building a strong body takes time. It takes dedication. But don't despair. It's the same patience and dedication you had as a child learning how to become strong enough to stand, walk, and play. If you did it once, you can certainly do it again.

We are a collection and an expression of the habits we keep. Our habits today shape the lives we'll have tomorrow. Having said that, the more you know about your habits, the better chance you have at changing them. In other words, to defeat our enemies, we must know our enemies. You have to know yourself!

3

REPETITION AND THE NERVOUS SYSTEM

"Don't make me pull this car over!"

—Every parent, ever

Habits are created by repetition. In fact, it's repetition that shapes our nervous system, and therefore the stories we live. Things we constantly hear, things we constantly do, and things we constantly experience all work together to sculpt our nervous system and create our habits, habits of thought and habits of action.

Good or bad, the repetitions of our day-to-day lives shape who we are. Our health, our emotions, even our relationships are all a result of the habits we keep.

There are varying statistics in research regarding how many days it takes to build a habit. Some researchers suggest it takes twenty-one days to build a habit. Others say twenty-eight days. New research indicates that it may take sixty-six days.[1] Regardless of how many days it takes to build a habit, two things are certain:

There is a first time for everything. Habits have a starting point, or a moment when an action or thought was born. This is true for both the habits you currently have and the habits you want to create.

A good habit can begin today. Habits are built by daily, consistent repetition, of a particular behavior, whether it is a behavior of thought or action. The habits you have are the habits you create through daily practice.

The point—whoever you are and whatever life you want to live—is a result, or will be the result of the repetitive decisions you make day in and day out. As far as your nervous system is concerned, you are what you do. If you understand this and you understand you were intended to be strong, then you can see how your habits were intended to be the vehicle for maintaining strength. To see how this is true, let's take a look at the nervous system.

---

[1]   http://www.ucl.ac.uk/news/news-articles/0908/09080401.

4

CARVED IN LIVING STONE

Your brain is plastic. No, it is not made of fossil fuels. It is *plastic,* capable of changing its structure and neural connections. In fact, it is now believed that every single action you do, and every thought you have, actually changes the structure of your brain in order for your brain to become more efficient.[2] So, every single thing you do shapes your brain in some way.[3]

Now, here's the crazy part: You are capable of an infinite number of thoughts and possibly an infinite number of movements. To be sure, every person ultimately has a finite amount of thoughts and movements while they exist on this earth, but there are no limits to the number of thoughts and movements a person can make while they're physically alive. My point in bringing this up is that if a person could have limitless thoughts and movements, and every single new thing a person does creates a new neural connection, then the amount of possible neural connections in the brain would be staggering. It is. Scientists now believe there

[2]   Norman Doidge, *The Brain that Changes Itself* (New York: The Penguin Group, 2007), p. xviii.
[3]   Norman Doidge, *The Brain that Changes Itself* (New York: The Penguin Group, 2007), p. 208.

are over several 100 trillion neural connections in the brain.[4] Just think how awesomely and wonderfully created you are. Your body is a glorious and miraculous masterpiece.

Anyway, everything about the brain and the body is made to be efficient. Like the body, the brain works off the "use it or lose it" principle. Conversely, the brain and body also work off the "use it and keep it" principle. This is where repetition allows the brain to change enough to create habits. Let's look at how this might work.

Learning a new skill changes the structure of your brain by creating new neural connections. Repetition of this new skill cements these neural connections in your brain[5], making the neural connections more efficient and requiring less thought. Eventually, the brain can go on autopilot when performing what *once* was a new skill because the neural connections for this activity become very efficient.

This process is how habits are formed. The first time you do something, whether it is an action or a thought, you create a change in your brain, or a new connection. The second time you do that same something makes that new connection a little bit stronger and a little more efficient. The thousandth time you do that same something, you create such a well-grooved connection, the brain forgets it was ever a new skill. You have made a very efficient neural connection that requires very little thought or energy. This can be both good and bad because the brain doesn't discriminate between good and bad habits. The brain only strives

---

[4] http://theastronomist.fieldofscience.com/2011/07/cubic-millimeter-of-your-brain.html.

[5] Norman Doidge, *The Brain that Changes Itself* (New York: The Penguin Group, 2007), p. 209.

to make itself efficient and good at what it does. Good or bad, pretty or ugly, habits are etched into your brain![6]

Now that we know habits are formed in the brain, the phrases *stuck in a rut, set in his ways*, and *force of habit* all make sense, and they all ring true. If you have a habit, you are stuck in a rut, a neuronal-circuit-rut grooved out somewhere inside your brain. You are indeed "set" in your ways and may literally perform actions out of a force of habit. This is called rigidity.[7] Anything you do that involves repetition—whether it be your career, your sport, your neurotic thoughts, even your bedtime routine—can lead to rigidity.[8]

We are literally creatures of habit. We are wired for efficiency. If it were not so, the brain would not so readily carve out our repeated actions and thoughts with well-grooved neural pathways. Being efficient is a matter of survival. The less energy the brain has to use to process our thoughts and movements, the more energy we will have to live and to survive.

For example, learning how to walk takes a lot of energy, both physically and mentally. This may be one reason babies take so many "rest breaks" and naps. Once the skill of walking is owned, it becomes effortless, physically and mentally. Yes, there is a caloric cost to walking, but it is an efficiently-used caloric cost. Think about it, you can walk for miles without thought or effort. But if you were just now learning how to walk, it would exhaust you. Now, replace walking with any new skill you have fought to learn, and remember how taxing it was. I used the words "fought to learn" because the brain is efficient, and it strives to remain

---

[6]   Norman Doidge, *The Brain that Changes Itself* (New York: The Penguin Group, 2007), p. 209.

[7]   Norman Doidge, *The Brain that Changes Itself* (New York: The Penguin Group, 2007), p. 242.

[8]   Norman Doidge, *The Brain that Changes Itself* (New York: The Penguin Group, 2007), p. 242.

that way. A new skill, or anything requiring new neural connections takes energy. Especially when the brain would rather be using the neural connections that it has already grooved so well.

We cannot fight being creatures of habit. That is how we are made. We are an expression of our thoughts and actions, both good and bad. But that is good news. If we are a collection of our habits, and our brains are good at building habits, we can create the habits we want to have. This will take work, mind you, and we may even have to fight for these new habits, but we are capable of creating the habits we desire. We can take what the brain does so well and use it to our advantage. We can trade less-desirable habits for most-desirable habits.

Yes, the habits we want to replace are well-grooved inside our brains, but the new habits we want to create will eventually become well-grooved too. Especially if we keep repeating those desired thoughts or actions. Not only that, but because of neuronal pruning,[9] our "bad" habits will become less efficient the less we use them. In other words, the brain does not reinforce neural connections for efficiency if those neural connections aren't being used. And, those unused neural connections, while they may still be there, will eventually become less and less efficient. You can weaken your bad habits by not participating in them. This is how most people actually weaken their good strength habits. They simply don't participate in them like they once did and as a consequence, their health fades.

Habits are created and weakened by simple addition. If you can add, you can change your habits. Before we get into how to change our habits, there's more you should know. Habits live inside your brain, but they can be manifested or expressed through your body. Remember, the body is like the brain in that it strives for efficiency.

---

[9] Sally Goddard Blythe, *The Well Balanced Child* (Stroud: Hawthorne Press, 2005), p. 23.

5

You've SAID Enough

Have you ever heard of the SAID principle? It stands for Specific Adaptation to Imposed Demands. The SAID principle states that the body will always adapt to exactly what it does.[10] Why does the body do this? Because the body loves efficiency. We are conservers of energy. Our bodies love to make the things we do easier for us to do. This is how we develop skills and habits. Our nervous system and body adapts to the stresses we place on them, and we eventually become good at doing whatever it is we're doing.

An example of the SAID principle is strength training. If you lift weights, your muscles get bigger and you get stronger. But did you also know your tendons get stronger, your bones become thicker, and your metabolism increases? These changes, along with others, are a result of the stresses that are placed on the body while strength training.

As we learned in the previous chapter, the SAID principle is demonstrated in our brains by the way our habits create efficient neural pathways to allow us to easily continue our habits. In other words, getting habitually stuck in a rut is a result of

---

[10]   http://en.wikipedia.org/wiki/SAID_principle.

the SAID principle taking place in your brain. The body always adapts to exactly what it does. Your brain, which is part of your body, adapts in the same way.

Because of the SAID principle, our habits physically live in our brains in the form of neural pathways. Habits can also physically live in our bodies as well in the form of postures, movements, and even respirations. Because the body is always adapting to exactly what it does, your body will also adapt to the habits you carry in your brain.

Did you know sitting is a habit? Whether you believe it's true or not, admit it, you are really good at sitting. You've had lots of practice, and your body has adapted to allow you to easily sit in the manner you do. Do you sit in front of a computer all day? Do you sit with your shoulders rounded forward? Do you keep your right hand elevated on your mouse for most of the day? When you stand up, are your shoulders still rounded forward? Is your right shoulder still slightly elevated from having your hand on your mouse? Are you still in your "computer posture," or are you standing tall with perfect posture? The body actually adapts so well to some things, like sitting, that it becomes difficult for us to do other things, like standing with good posture.

Keep in mind that your body strives to be efficient. Or, to put it another way, your body strives to be perfect at what it does. To continue with our sitting example, years of sitting with poor posture could be an impetus for the body to change its structure to allow the body to hold that sitting position effortlessly. To do this, the body may get rid of muscle mass that is not needed, it may increase fascia tension and thickness along the spine to help hold that rounded thoracic curve better, and it may cause some bone and joint deterioration. You may even lose the coordination for everyday things like running, skipping, or even walking, because you simply don't need these skills if all you do, for most of the day, is sit. Remember the parable at the beginning of the chapter?

"But from those who do nothing, even what little they have will be taken away."—Matthew 25:29

This is neural pruning in action. If you don't use it, you lose it.

The message here is that your habits, your lifestyle, and your routines can and will be expressed by your body. And don't forget, every single thing you do, in order for you to do it well, creates neural pathways inside your brain to support your activities. Habits seem to become a self-sustaining cycle in that respect. The brain and the body both make it easy for you to continue doing the things that you do, and they support each other in doing so. This is what makes lifelong habits challenging to change. They've become well-engrained in both the body and the brain.

However, all hope is not lost. If anything, understanding how habits are formed in the brain and the body should create a surge of hope that new habits and tendencies can be created as well. The very process that allowed us to create the habits we have also allows us to change the habits we don't want, or exchange them with new ones.

Now that we understand habits a little better, we need to understand where they come from.

6

TO BE OR NOT TO BE

"You must choose. But choose wisely."

—Grail Knight's character in
Indiana Jones and the Last Crusade

Our habits are a result of our choices.

The body you have is the body you've earned or, rather, chosen. This can be a hard slap of reality. If you're in good health, you've earned it! Conversely, if you're in poor health, well, you've earned that too. To be clear, I am only referring to our bodies being a result of our choices and lifestyles. There are some things we don't choose, like injurious accidents, birth defects, or any number of other physical limitations. Still, even within these circumstances, habits are chosen. Whether we want to admit it or not, as adults, we choose our habits. Once we've chosen our habits, they become real, physical changes inside our bodies and brains. Therefore, we choose the bodies we have.

The power of choice determines our habits. It is the power of choice that determines who we are. Choice is perhaps the most powerful weapon that mankind can wield. It is choice that leads to world wars, choice that leads to riotous destruction, and choice that leads to the dinner you decide to eat tonight. Thankfully, it is also choice that leads to creating a new life, choice that leads to buying a coat for someone in need, and choice that leads to going for a walk in the park. Choice is powerful. It is your weapon. You are the one who takes aim.

With your weapon of choice (pun intended), you've decided what habits you created. So, to say it again, the body you have is the body you have chosen. In other words, you are not the victim. You are the perpetrator of your current situation.

I know what you're thinking. There are other factors involved in a person's life, factors like culture, the environment, and genetics. You are correct. Let us look at genetics as an example. It's true you can't choose the genes that you're born with. Your parents determine your genes, but did you know you have a choice on how those genes are expressed? I'm not saying you can choose to change your brown eyes to blue, but you can make lifestyle choices that either silence or amplify the expression of your genes![11] This is fantastic news! You don't necessarily have to be a victim of your genetics!

Your genes may not be the self-fulfilling prophecy tellers they're made out to be. If you don't believe me, let's look at a real world example. Take a pair of identical twins. They're genetically identical. They're clones. Now let's assume that they grow up in the same environment and share the same culture. After all, they are twins! If their genes truly determined how they will end up in life, they should end up exactly the same at age forty. But this won't necessarily be the case at all. One twin could make a lifetime of healthy choices and become the picture of health and good living. The other twin could make a lifetime of

---

[11] Todd Harnagan, *Wellness, the 5 Essential Elements* (New York: Gallup Press) p. 74.

not-so-healthy choices and end up obese, sickly, or even dead. It is the power of choice that makes the difference, not genetics.

You can absolutely effect how your genes are expressed through the choices you make. Even wilder than that, biologists have actually discovered a new phenomenon know as "epigenetic inheritance" that indicates the life choices you make today could even influence the genes you pass on to your children and your grandchildren![12] How awesome is that? Your choices may even determine the genes that you pass down to future generations! Do you see what I mean? Choice is extremely powerful.

When it comes to establishing healthy habits and building the strength your body was meant to have, it all hinges on the choices you make. In life we accumulate choices. You can make and accumulate positive choices—choices that positively effect the outcome of your health and life, or you can make negative choices—choices that negatively influence the outcome of your health and life. The trick is to make more positive choices than negative ones.

You decide if you honor your design by moving often. You decide if you eat vegetables. You decide if you get to bed by 10:00 pm. You get the point, right? The choice is yours when it comes to having the health you desire. We are a collection of the choices we make. We are a collection of the habits we create. We choose what neural connections we cement inside our brains as well as the ones we weaken.

And, we can change one choice at a time, one day at a time. Rome wasn't built in a day, and neither were you. The body you've chosen took time to build. The body you want to have will take time to build as well.

---

[12] Anderson and Neupert, *Pressing Reset: Original Strength Reloaded* (Fuquay-Varina: Font Publishing).

7

YOU ARE WHAT
YOU THINK

*"…Guard your heart above all else,
for it determines the course of your life….."*

—Psalm 4:23

The more you think the same thoughts, the more you cement those neural connections and they can become engrained and efficient. Think about this for a second, the thoughts you keep in your head, the ones you keep thinking, actually become real physical connections in your brain. They have physical representations, they take up space, inside your brain. Isn't that amazing?

Here's a question for you: What are you thinking?

What thoughts do you keep in your head? I ask because thoughts don't just become real connections in your brain, they become real expressions in your body and in your life. Your thoughts can determine the course of your health.

Have you ever met a hypochondriac? Are they always sick? Why do you think that is? Because they keep thinking they're going to get sick, and they do. Let's look at someone else. Have you ever met a person who always thinks fearful thoughts? Maybe they are afraid of getting fired or something. Visualize them in your mind. What does their posture look like? Do they stand tall and strong, or do they slump and keep their head down? Do they appear calm and pleasant? Or do they breathe shallow and seem stressed or frantic? They may never get fired, but the fear of getting fired likely manifests in the person's body. The body expresses what the mind is thinking.

Think of all the different types of people there are in the world. There are optimists, pessimists. There are those who are happy, angry, brave, scared, strong-willed, wishy-washy. What do their bodies typically look like in your mind's eye? Do their postures and expressions match their way of thinking? More than likely, they do.

Your brain is powerful. Again, your thoughts and expectations will determine your outcome. People live according to their beliefs. Thoughts of sickness and weakness produce brokenness. Thoughts of health and strength produce resiliency. This happens not only because thoughts actually change the shape of the brain, but also because thoughts become beliefs. When you believe something because it is so engrained inside of your head, it becomes your reality.

This is why it is so important to guard your thoughts. If you're not thinking thoughts of health and strength, you won't have them, regardless of whether or not you want them. For example, a person can want to be in good health and live a long life, but they may be constantly thinking they will die before they are fifty because, after all, heart disease runs in their family. It is hard to walk around in strength when your brain is conceiving and building neural pathways that say you are going to die before you turn fifty.

As an adult, the path to strength and health starts in your mind. It starts with your thoughts. You must gain control of your thoughts and start thinking thoughts of health, strength, and resiliency. You mustn't allow thoughts of weakness, sickness, and fear to invade your brain.

Such thoughts are traps. They increase your stress. Increased stress leads to disease.

You were created to be strong. Choose to be strong.

8

THE ROOTS OF STRENGTH

"I know kung fu."

—Neo's character from *The Matrix*

You have an original operating system inside of you, firmware, if you will. Inside your original operating system, you have been programmed to be strong. When you were a child, you executed this program, you carried out the movements embedded in the program, and day by day through repetition, you became strong. You carved out these movements in your brain, through neuroplasticity, and you became efficient at executing them both, inside your nervous system and with your body. This is how you established your foundation of strength, your reflexive strength.

Reflexive strength is the strength upon which your body establishes all movement and ability. It is the strength that helps your body anticipate movement before it even happens, it is the strength that allows your body to react to movement imposed on it, and it is the strength that keeps you from becoming weak or injured. Movement by movement (habit by habit), you established reflexive strength along with new neural connections allowing you to build even more strength. Eventually, you became strong enough to stand, to walk, to climb, to run, to be.

It doesn't really matter what the current state of your body is. You were designed, preprogrammed, to be amazingly strong. Though you may not be a child anymore and some of the neural connections you built so diligently may have faded or become dull, your original operating system is still inside of you. If you tap back into your original operating system, if you revisit the simple movements designed to give you the foundation of strength, you can return your body back to its intended design. In other words, you can become strong and healthy through the simple movements you made as a child. Once you firmly reestablish these movements back into your nervous system, they again become your foundation to continue to progress and increase your health even more.

This may sound like a stretch, and may take a leap of faith, but if you reset your ways and remember how you once moved as a child, you can restore the strength you were designed to have.

Children are programmed to move, so their thoughts really don't get in the way of their strength development. They breathe the way they were designed, they keep their heads level with the horizon through reflexes and constant effort, and they learn how to move across the floor, usually driven by curiosity. The point is, a child is constantly trying to learn to move. When they tire, they rest, but then they're right back at it. They have a determination most adults have lost sight of. They also have an advantage: They don't have any concept of failure and they haven't learned how to be afraid. Like I said, their thoughts don't get in the way of their development.

In the next few sections, I'm going to take you through the big five RESETS, as seen in the book *Pressing Reset: Original Strength*

Reloaded[13]. These are the developmental movements children use to develop immense strength and resiliency. This will be just a brief overview of these movements, but presented with a slightly different perspective than what's presented in *Pressing Reset*.

If you're unfamiliar with these RESETs, think of them like reset buttons for the body. To perform these movements once in a while is good, but it won't produce the habits of strength you want. What you want, is to develop habitual strength—the strength you can't lose because you're continually engaging in your original design, your original operating system, building and solidifying strong neural connections and reflexes throughout your entire nervous system, thus building and solidifying reflexive strength throughout your entire body. The deeper your foundation of reflexive strength, the deeper its roots—and the healthier and more capable your body becomes.

As we explore the big five RESETS, keep in mind most of these movements were once habits of yours. They created a solid foundation of reflexive strength, from which you layered more and more strength and became more and more capable. At least, once upon a time, it was true.

---

[13] Anderson and Neupert, *Pressing Reset: Original Strength Reloaded* (Fuquay-Varina: Font Publishing).

9

CLOSE YOUR MOUTH

Has anyone ever told you to close your mouth when you chew your food? I'm sure most of us, at some point, have heard this. After all, it is good manners. Remember those? What about breathing? Has anyone ever told you to close your mouth when you breathe? No, it's not necessarily a manners issue, but it could be a huge strength issue.

Once upon a time, you were an obligate nasal breather. This means every breath you made was through your nasal passages - unless they were clogged or you were crying. Children breathe through their nose for the first three months of their lives, and they primarily breathe through their nose past the first six months of their lives.[14] Children also breathe deep into their bellies by using their diaphragm, their breathing muscle. (It's still your breathing muscle.). If a baby starts breathing up in their chest and neck, through their mouths, they are probably sick and their breathing is significantly compromised.

Habitually speaking, as a child, you were a very good diaphragmatic, nasal breather. A baby less than six months old typically

---

[14]   http://www.livestrong.com/article/274704-mouth-breathing-in-infants/.

breathes between thirty to sixty breaths per minute.[15] For example, let's just say a baby breathes forty-five breaths per minute. There are 1,140 minutes in a day and there are roughly thirty days in a month. So, If a baby is an obligatory nasal breather for the first three months of life, they could potentially take 1,944,000 diaphragmatic, nasal breaths. By six months of age, a baby would probably be around 3.5 million diaphragmatic nasal breaths. That's a pretty efficient neural pathway, wouldn't you think?

Every breath you take should be a breath of strength. You were designed to be a "big belly" nasal breather throughout your entire life. You executed millions of repetitions (breaths) in an effort to establish this pattern (habit). Breathing through your nose, deep into your belly, is the most simple, yet powerful secret to strength and health. In fact, it is actually reflexive core training. One of the best ways to protect your spine and strengthen your center is to breathe with your diaphragm. A solid center is the key to strength.

Through a course of varying events, for one reason or another, many adults change or override their default breathing pattern through practicing another way to breathe. Maybe they breathe through their mouths or maybe they breathe up into their chests and necks. Many times, they do both. It can start as simple as a non-optimal breath here and there, and then it becomes more and more executed. Eventually, it becomes a habit. Habits and neural pathways are a game of numbers. It only takes doing something once to create a new neural pathway, or a new option. Do it several thousand times, and your create a new normal.

But wait, how can such an engrained breathing pattern be overturned so easily? After all, the young baby performed over 3 million diaphragmatic breaths by the time they were six months old. Does an adult somehow flip a switch and perform 4 million

---

[15]   http://www.webmd.com/children/normal-breathing-rates-for-children.

breaths to establish a new, more powerful habit than the one we were programmed with?

Maybe. Remember, the baby doesn't know fear or failure. But as we grow, we begin to learn such things. Emotions get tied to our movements and our actions. Emotions can be a powerful weight that shifts the "habit scales" faster than numbers alone. There is a saying that "Nerves that fire together, wire together." Emotional, traumatic events in our lives can become wired to our movements and our patterns, and sometimes it only has to happen once. Emotional trauma (fear, terror, failure, stress, sadness) can be powerful multipliers when it comes to developing a habit we don't want. Think of it this way: a simple movement can "scratch" or "etch" a new neural connection into your brain. A movement associated with trauma can "puncture" neural connections into your brain, or scar you. This is an oversimplification, but I hope it makes the point.

This is another reason why it's so important to have deeply engrained patterns and habits we actually do want. If they are carved deep enough, even if they are hijacked by emotional events, we can return to them with a little effort. I know for certain you've got at least 3 million diaphragmatic, nasal breaths in your brain somewhere. I'm betting we can find them and dust them off.

Another secret of breathing with the diaphragm is, it helps control your thoughts. When we breathe like we were designed, the body operates in "rest and digest" mode. It's at peace, there's no emergency, the adrenaline alarms aren't going off and the brain can think soberly, clearly, and rationally. Conversely, when we live in a perpetual emergency because we are breathing with our emergency muscles, stress is in the air and it can permeate our ability to think, focus, and be. Children seem pretty stress-free, don't they? They're living examples of how we're all supposed to be.

The point is breathing with the diaphragm is the one habit, the one "movement" we should make the greatest effort to regain. This one habit alone can change your life for the better.

So, how are you supposed to breathe?

Close your mouth, place your tongue on the roof of your mouth, breathe into your nose and pull air down into your belly. Your belly should expand, but so should your sides and lower back. Breathing is a full "core-expanding" movement.

Simply spending five to ten minutes a day practicing this can help the brain remember and restore this movement back to your default operating mode. Please note, this may not be as easy as you think. For some, diaphragmatic breathing may be a challenge, especially if it's been a long while since the days of your childhood.

A great way to practice is to lie on the floor in a position of comfort and then breathe. Ideally, you want to be able to breathe with your diaphragm in every single position you can put your body in, but for now, let's practice in a position you enjoy. As you get comfortable breathing with your diaphragm, you can practice while sitting at your desk, while driving, while walking, and even while running. Those are progressions, but they're attainable. It's your design to breathe this way.

Do this every day:

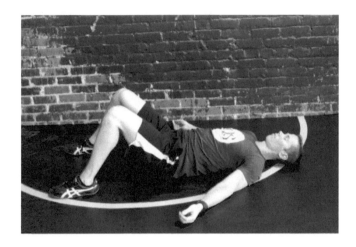

- Close your mouth.
- Put your tongue on the roof of your mouth.
- Breathe deep into your belly through your nose.

Strength starts here. Practice this five to ten minutes each day.

This is ridiculously easy strength training. It really is.

10

BIG HEADS = STRONG BODIES

Another habit you once had, was keeping your head level with the horizon. You still have this ability, but you probably try to override it more than you reinforce it. In today's world of smartphones and social awkwardness, many people tend to hold their heads down and don't walk around with the crown of their heads held high to the sky. People tend not to move their heads around anymore either. While our heads sit on a swivel, it is rare to see people really use that swivel anymore. Yes, today's adults have, literally, forgotten how to use their heads. But it is the ability to move the head, to control the head as we all once did, that's a major key, if not *the* key, to building and restoring strength.

You were born with the righting reflex built into your nervous system. The righting reflex is basically a reflex designed to keep your head level with the horizon. When you were a child, this reflex caused you to strengthen your entire body through holding your head up and setting your gaze level with the horizon. You built amazing strength through learning how to hold your head up and then mastering the movements of your head.

If you consider that a baby's head is one-fourth the size of their body and it weighs roughly 30 percent as much as their entire body, mastering head control is the ultimate ingredient in strength training. It is also the ultimate necessity. Without head control, your balance, posture, and coordination will always be lacking.[16]

Let's look at the size of a baby's head again. Today, the average adult male weighs about 190 pounds.[17] At this weight, if the average adult male, had a baby's head, it would weigh about fifty-seven pounds! Can you imagine walking around with a fifty-seven-pound head? Can you imagine how strong you would become learning how to move around with a head that weighed that much? A child learns, through a decent supply of bumps and bruises, how to master and control their proportionately large and heavy head. The movements of their head are tied to every muscle in their body. Learning to balance, turn, lift, and level their head is like strength training and fine-tuning all the muscles in their body.

As adults, our heads are only about one-eighth the size of our body and weigh between eight to twelve pounds. Nowhere near as large or heavy as a child's, relative to our own body size, yet head control or mastery is something that has slipped away from us.

Like breathing, we acquired several repetitions of head control in the form of practice, learning, and time as children. We can regain head control again by relearning how to move our heads. We start this process the same way we did as children: we just have to get down on the floor (or lay down). Lying down and learning how to lift and move the head is a great way to regain control of our head movements and reinforce the wonderful

---

[16] Sally Goddard Blythe, The Well Balanced Child - balance posture coordination.

[17] http://pediatrics.about.com/cs/growthcharts2/f/avg_wt_male.htm.

neural connections in our brains, along with the reflexive muscular connections that run throughout our bodies.

Head nods and rotations are an easy way to build the kind of strength that removes the limitations from the body. Done consistently, done in such a way that head control—moving your head as per your original operating system—becomes part of your everyday life. Balance, posture, and coordination are restored, and mobility and strength are allowed to be fully expressed. Having head control is a habit that leads to real strength.

Do this every day:

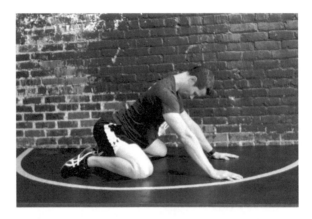

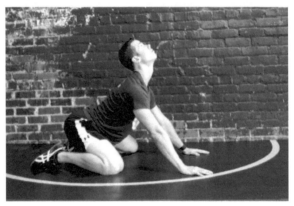

- Get on all fours.
- Look up as high as you can.
- Lead with your eyes.
- Lower you chin to your chest.
- Next, rotate your head around from side to side, as if trying to look at your own feet.
- Lead with your eyes.

You can do this for reps, or simply do this for two to three minutes. Go slow, don't move into pain, and don't make yourself dizzy.

11

FLOWING STRENGTH

We should all move gracefully. Many of us once did. Graceful movement comes from engaging in movement on a regular basis. It also comes from the ability to move our joints the way they were designed to move. When you were a child, more than likely, you spent a great deal of time on the floor until you learned how to walk. Back then, you learned the rules and the law of the Big G: gravity. Crashing a noggin into the floor can be a great teacher. Learning how to wage war against your invisible nemesis made you stronger. Fighting gravity is how you learned to move your body, piece by piece and part by part, until your whole body flowed with ease.

It is this ability to flow like an ocean wave that allows your body to express the beautiful strength you were designed to have. Grace might not be your middle name, but there was a time when it probably should have been.

Rolling on the floor is primarily where you developed the ability to flow as a child. If you have ever witnessed a child roll over, you will see a flowing, segmental (piece-by-piece) roll. If you contrast that with the way most adults roll, you will see a completely different story. Many adults roll over as one piece; they look like a stiff log. They have unlearned how to segment their body freely and they don't really spend too much time allowing their spines to rotate. Thus, they lose their ability to flow.

Remembering how to roll—vertebrae by vertebrae—is where we restore our grace and flow. It is also where we start to nurture and lubricate our spines while at the same time restoring our reflexive strength. If we can help our brains remember how to roll our bodies with fluidity, then all the other movements we engage in will start to ooze fluidity. Walking will start to look like a poetic dance instead of a Frankenstein-created movement. Fluid movement is the gateway for optimal strength to be expressed. It is the difference between driving a golf ball seventy-five yards and driving one 300 yards. It is also the difference between falling apart at age thirty and living strong and capable at age eighty. The better you flow, the further you will go.

Rolling just a few minutes a day can do wonders for the health of your spine, your brain, your body, and your strength. Rolling also requires head control, and it continues to activate and strengthen your vestibular system similar to the head nods mentioned above. Therefore rolling is another great way to restore and improve balance, posture, and coordination.

Let's look at an easy way to remember how to roll. Lie on your back with your hands overhead. Keeping your head on the floor, look to your left and rotate your head to your left. Take your right leg, bend your knee, and reach across your body with your knee as if trying to roll your hip over. Now take your right arm and reach in across your body. Allow your head to lift up from the floor as you reach. You should easily roll to your left side. (It may help tremendously to place a shiny red ball or a smart phone by your side to reach for.) This rotates your spine from your hips all the way up to your head.

To unroll, simply reverse the process. Return your right arm back to where you had it and lower your head back down to the floor. Return your right leg to where it started, and rotate your head back to the center. Now repeat the same sequence by rolling onto your right side. This rotates your spine from your head all the way back down to your hips.

This is a similar roll most babies flow in and out of, but it is also a little different. Your limbs are a little longer, and your head is a little smaller, but this is a great and easy way to start remembering how to roll and rotate as it allows your brain to learn how to let pieces of your body begin to segment and flow. Once you begin to flow in and out of this roll, you can easily learn how to roll from your back to your belly and from your belly to your back.

Your rolling patterns live in your brain. By spending time rolling, you can find them, restore them and strengthen them. If you can become consistent and return rolling to your habitual movement repertoire, you will begin to flow with strength and power.

Do this every day:

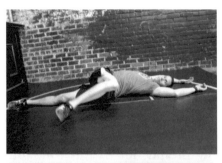

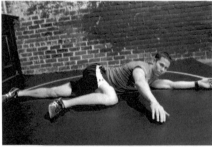

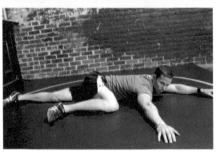

- Lie on your back with your arms overhead.
- Look left and rotate your head.
- Reach across your body with your right leg.
- Reach across your body with your right arm and roll to your side.
- Pick up your head as you reach.
- Reverse the process and then repeat the steps to your right side.

Spend about three minutes each day rolling on the floor. Roll back and forth from side to side. This is a great way to mobilize your spine and regain fluid movement throughout your body.

12

ARTICULATORS, ASSEMBLE!

Chances are you went from the lifestyle of moving, the habit of moving all the time to a lifestyle of stillness. Children are always moving, exploring, playing, and learning with and through their bodies. Learning how to move is what assimilates the body into one being. It assimilates the whole of you, not just your physical attributes but it also assimilates your senses. Movement teaches the brain depth perception. Movement sharpens your sense of touch, balance, control, and even your sense of judgment. How do you know how to throw a football at a moving target? How does your brain know how to judge how hard to throw, how far to lead the target, how to coordinate the timing of your throw and the speed of the target to anticipate the perfect placement of the football? The brain learns all of this through the body's attempts to learn how to move.

Movement coordinates and integrates all of you. One movement in particular does a fantastic job of this: rocking.

Rocking, swaying, and swinging have been tactics used by man throughout centuries to calm and nurture children. Children preparing their bodies and minds for movements use rocking, swaying, and swinging too. Before they crawl, babies often get up on their hands and knees and rock back and forth. As they do this, they often smile and giggle.

Rocking is a movement—and habit—you want to reintegrate into your life. It's probably the simplest and easiest mobility and strength-training movement you possess. Yes, getting on your hands and knees, rocking back and forth, is strength training. If you do it often enough, you will start to feel like you have a new body.

Your body has numerous synovial joints and numerous muscles that facilitate the movements of these joints. Rocking integrates most of them into your brain and prepares your body for movement. You have stabilizing muscles and muscles called prime movers. Rocking teaches your stabilizers how to stabilize your joints when they should be stable and how to allow the prime movers to move your joints when they should move. When your stabilizers and your prime movers know their roles and when your nervous system is well tuned and sharp, your body is free to express the mobility and strength it is designed to have.

There's a simple explanation. Rocking teaches your muscles how to coordinate their roles and responsibilities, and it teaches your brain how to move your joints so you can move fluidly and with grace. In this respect, rocking is an extension of rolling. Do you see how simple movements build upon each other to establish a foundation of strength?

Another wonderful benefit to rocking is that it builds good posture, and it reflexively sets and reveals the posture we should have. As we are rocking, our spinal stabilizers learn how to reflexively stabilize our spine. This is where we build the natural curves of our spine and teach our vertebrae how to respond to movement. This is why you should rock. If for no other reason, it helps rebuild and restore your posture. In order to be strong and healthy, to resist and endure the wiles of life's activities, you need and want to have optimal, reflexively-sharp posture.

Spending a little time rocking every day will start to make you feel new. You will begin to stand taller, move better, feel better, and the small things in life will suddenly become easier.

Do this every day:

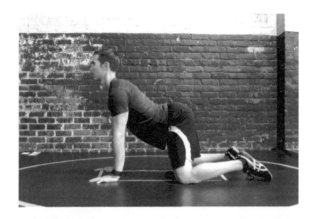

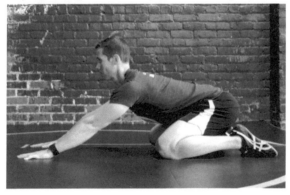

- Get on your hands and knees.
- Hold your head up (look at the horizon).
- Keep a proud chest, and push your butt back towards your feet.
- Don't let your spine round like a bridge. Keep it flat by holding a proud chest.

You can rock back and forth several times a day for twenty or more reps. It will take all of thirty seconds. You can also spend a minute or two here and there and rock while playing with different speeds and foot positions. It's easy, it doesn't take long, and the return is tremendous.

If you can't get down on the floor, do this on a bed, or use pillows if your knees are tender. Find a way to rock. Don't move into pain, but persist in discovering a way to remember how to do this motion. It really is powerful.

13

MARCH ACROSS TO THE OTHER SIDE

Perhaps that greatest habit we all need to regain is moving from point A to point B. As kids we spent most of our time on the floor getting strong enough to be able to get across the floor. Once kids learn how to crawl and walk, there is almost no holding them back from moving forward into new territories and adventures.

It's this process of strengthening and moving through the gait cycle that develops the foundation of our reflexive strength. It builds our brain, sharpens our nervous system (makes it fast, alert, and efficient), and it strengthens our bodies (our fascia, ligaments, tendons, bones, and muscles, heart, lungs, blood vessels—all of it).

The one thing we were all created to do, without any question, is walk. We were designed to move from one place to another by using all four of our limbs, on a very regular, consistent basis. Walking, true walking, was the vehicle that would keep our brains healthy, our nervous system sharp, and our bodies strong. It would constantly reinforce our foundation of strength, allowing us to build and add to our structure effectively. A strong foundation will support almost any structure and a weak foundation will be the demise of even the strongest structure.

Again, as infants, we all spent the majority of our time learning how to move to become strong enough to walk. Then, we spent the majority of our time moving: walking, running, skipping, and playing. Everything we did deepened our roots, our foundation, and we became resilient through the driven, habitual movements that we made. I use the word "driven" for a reason. There is a drive in all of us to move. We once followed it. Most of us have been taught how to override it and suppress it, but the drive is still inside of us somewhere. It is our design to move and to be strong. There is a drive behind the design. Can you find it again?

I am not saying that walking will make you a powerlifting champion. What I am saying is that by engaging your true gait pattern, with all four limbs, whether by crawling, marching, walking, or running, will start to rebuild your foundation of reflexive strength enabling your to become absolutely as strong as you would hope to be. Four-limb locomotion will tie your body together (think mind, brain, nerves, connections, muscles, systems) and allow you to express your potential. It is worth uncovering the drive behind the design and following that drive to constant engagement.

Your strength lives in the simplicity of your design. It's brilliant.

Some of you reading this might significantly benefit from learning how to crawl again. Relearning to crawl can be miraculous for many people in the way in which it leads to the restoration of the body. To this end, I offer the marching cross-crawl.

Marching is kind of like crawling while standing. It's deliberate in that, much like crawling, all four limbs are brought into play. Cross-crawls are extremely powerful in that they engage, much like crawling does, both hemispheres of the brain and almost anyone, regardless of their condition can perform them. When you combine the march with a cross-crawl, it's like double-dipping.

You're engaging in two deliberate exercises at the same time, and both strengthen your brain and your body. This is an easy way to start restoring your reflexive foundation of strength. It can be done anywhere, and it doesn't have to take a great deal of time. It's perhaps the simplest thing you can do to yield the greatest results.

The marching cross-crawl is basically just the normal cross-crawl except the arms move more deliberately from flexion to extension. If you can, march while touching your opposite elbow to your knee. If this is an impossibility for now, touch your opposite forearm to your knee. If this is still a dream, march while touching your opposite hand to your knee. Whichever way you do it, make sure the back swinging arm reaches back from the shoulder and actually moves your hand back past the plane of your back.

Do this every day:

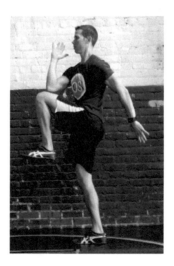

- Keep your eyes looking forward.
- Swing your arms from the shoulders.
- Touch your elbow to your opposite knee.
- Land softly on the balls of your feet.
- March with purpose.

You can march for twenty cross-crawl touches here and there throughout the day, or you can simply march for two to three minutes at a time. This is an invigorating movement snack!

14

ALL THE RIGHT MOVES

I see men like trees, walking.

—Mark 8:24

We just took a look at variations of the big five RESETS within the original strength movement restoration system. The RESETS are movements you should, without thought, do. While you might think of them as habitual movements, in truth, they're really deeper than habit. They "came with the frame" so to speak. You were preprogrammed with them and meant to engage in them throughout your life in some fashion. These RESETS are the foundation, or roots, of your strength.

Once that foundation has been laid, there are other movements your body was designed to perform day in and day out, on a regular, consistent basis. It is these other movements that build your structure. These are the movements worth building into habits. As we discuss these movements, notice how the RESETS underlay them. That is to say, these movements overlap and progress from the RESETS in many ways.

Famous strength coach and teacher, Dan John, teaches there are five human movements that everyone should do: squat, hinge, push, pull, and carry. If you study how the human body is designed, these movements are apparent. There is another movement I like to add to Dan's list: get-ups—simply getting up from the floor to standing. When you are ninety-nine years old, having the ability to easily get up from the floor is invaluable.

These six movements, and all their variations, build the structure of strength from which we were all designed to live. If the foundation, or the root, of the body is deep enough from moving through the RESETS, these movements can potentially become RESETS in themselves, continuing to keep the nervous system healthy. They can make the body "sharper," not just stronger.

The body was designed to move in and through these movements, their variations and their combinations. Wherever the body is, these movements should be available. What I mean by this is you don't need a health club membership to engage in these movements. They are available no matter where you are. However, if you want to add significant load to some of these movements, then a health club membership may be more cost and space effective than buying a great deal of equipment. Having said that, as long as you are willing to move your body, you can get as strong as you want to be with your own body, the resources available around you, and very little investment, other than time.

Let's take a quick look at these movements and discuss how they benefit our strength. Keep in mind, if you ever decide to engage in these movements, or any movements discussed in this book, there are four rules you must follow:

1. **Don't move into pain.** Deliberately doing something that hurts is not beneficial to your overall health and strength, and it may be detrimental to your strength.

2. **Start where you are.** We all bring different bodies and histories to the table when it comes to how we move. Whatever your past, whatever your current state, you are where you are. Start here. Start at now. Start.

3. **Use what you have.** Use your resources to your advantage. You have a body, use it as it allows you. Do you have ten spare minutes in your day to move? Use it. Do you only have floor space enough to do pushups? Great. You have all the space you need to become strong and powerful. Don't see limits. See what you have.

4. **Do what you can do.** You and I have different bodies. Our capabilities are probably different. You should seek to do what you are capable of doing, not what someone else is capable of doing. It is okay to be inspired by what others do, but don't try to do what they do if your isn't ready to do it. Be patient. Do what you can do. In time, as you become more capable, you will be able to do more

Okay, those are the rules, here are the movements:

The Squat

One of the very first movements you learned to do when you were learning to get on your feet and stand is the squat. It's one of the most foundational movement patterns of the human body. It is a way we get down to the ground, a way we get up from the ground, and it is a way we sit (or it once was) while on two feet.

The squat is also perhaps the most popular exercise in the strength training and fitness world. The squat is typically done on two feet side-by-side, and is performed by lowering the body towards the ground and "sitting" in between the legs.

In the strength training world, there are numerous variations of the squat. These variations generally have to do with where the load is placed, if any, and how the feet are positioned. The squat can also be done with staggered feet, or even on one foot.

There is always a debate about how low should a person squat. The depth of a squat depends on your intention. If you're trying to get down to the floor, or "sit" while on your feet, then you may want to be able to squat with your "butt to grass" or butt to calves, like a child does. Children are generally at rest when sitting in this position. If you want to rest while in a squat, this may be the best position.

Your optimal squat depth may be much different from mine. Maybe your squat depth is the depth that allows you to move pain free. Maybe your depth is the depth that your body will actually let you move. Maybe, as you continue to move and deepen your movement foundation, your depth next week will be much different than your depth today. Your squat depth is very dependent on you. Do what you can do—with control. Don't "fall" into a squat and bounce in it at the bottom. Pull yourself down, or lower yourself down, with strength. Don't fret about what you can't do. Enjoy what you can do.

The Hinge

Another foundational movement pattern to be enjoyed by us is the hinge. The hinge is done by bending at your hips. Imagine reaching down to touch your toes. That is hinging. It can be done on stiff, straight legs, or soft, bent knees. Hinging is something we might do to pick something up off the ground. Children often hinge to stand from the ground and they will also hinge when they're trying to pick something up that's too heavy for them to rise up from a squat. Some common names for the hinge in the exercise world are deadlifts, good mornings, and swings. Hinging can be done on two legs or on one leg. Single legged hinging is a wonderful way to hone in balance and refine strength.

For the purposes of this book, if you engage in picking objects up from the ground via hinging, keep your head (your gaze) on the horizon, keep your chest up and your back flat, much like the posture discussed in rocking from the previous chapter.

The Push

You were made to push things. Initially, as a child, you learned to push the world away from your chest. Pushing yourself up from the floor to crawl, and then crawling are examples of horizontal pushing. Horizontal pushing is a great way to keep things at arms length and protect yourself. Pushups, punches, and bench presses are all examples of pushing.

You are also capable of pushing things away from your torso laterally. In football, a stiff arm is a great example of a powerful lateral push. Pressing anything overhead as well as handstands and pushups are examples of vertical pushing.

Pushing objects, or pushing yourself away from objects, is a great way to add strength to your structure.

The Pull

Like the push, pulling can be done horizontally, laterally, or vertically. Pulling is simply pulling something towards you or pulling yourself towards something. Climbing and hanging is a great example of pulling with the arms. Tug of war is another great example. In today's world, even in the exercise and fitness world, pulling is often imbalanced from pushing. That is, most people seem to be better at pushing than pulling. There are many reasons for this. The biggest reason being that most of us simply don't get out and move as we were designed. Whatever the reason, a strong backside, is crucial for overall strength and health. In fact, our modern world was built on the backs of strong men and women.

Carries

This leads us to Dan's last big movement. Carries are essentially moving your body, with or without an external load, from one place to another. At its simplest form, a carry can be crawling or walking, engaging in your gait pattern, and moving your own bodyweight. From there, a carry could be moving any load, either on your body, against your body, or behind your body from one place to another.

It's my belief that carries are the secret to building Superman strength. In other words, engaging in the gait pattern, with and without external loads, is the secret sauce to building a body that's strong enough to last a lifetime worth living.

Carries are extremely simple to implement into your day. The intensity can easily be increased or decreased depending on your needs. You can carry for distance, time, speed or direction. You can carry on all fours or on two feet. There are so many wonderful variables to play with here.

I cannot stress the value of carries enough. If you only engaged in one structure-building, strength-building activity mentioned in this book, carry something and cover some distance—and do it often.

15

GET-UPS

"Well, which is it, young feller? You want I should freeze or get down on the ground? Mean to say, if'n I freeze, I can't rightly drop. And if'n I drop, I'm a-gonna be in motion."

—Feisty Hayseed's character in *Raising Arizona*

I separated get-ups from other movements for a couple of reasons. They aren't really part of Dan John's five human movements, and I think they deserve extra attention.

Get-ups can be any means or method from getting up from the floor or ground. There are specific get-ups like the Turkish get-up, a wonderful movement that entails standing up from the floor while holding a weight overhead. Get-ups can be done with bodyweight, sandbags, kids, dogs, dumbbells, and barbells. And, get-ups can be done creatively, in any way you can think of combined with whatever ways your body will allow you to move. Done frequently enough and with enough creativity, get-ups can become a RESET, as they can actually encompass each of the big five RESETs mentioned above. Yes, getting up and down from the floor can make your body stronger and more resilient.

In recent years, there have even been studies linking life expectancy with ease of effort, which one can rise up from the floor.[18] The gist of the studies is the easier you can get down and up from the floor, the longer you will live and less likely you are to have health issues.

Another reason you want to be able to easily get up from the floor is because this simple ability can set you free from fear. In some of my sobering experiences as a firefighter, I have been on emergency calls in which individuals had somehow found themselves on the floor, by falling or otherwise, and they couldn't get up. In some of these responses the individual had been on the floor for days, waiting for someone to find them. In others, they were able to get to a phone and call for help. It's no wonder some people are afraid to get down on the floor. It could mean disaster, but it shouldn't.

As a child, by learning how to move around on the floor, you once built and established all the strength you needed to conquer life. You can do the same thing again today, no matter how old you are. Learning to move around by getting up and down from the floor can absolutely restore the strength you need to conquer life again. It's just a matter of taking the time to explore the floor with get-ups.

The most important thing about get-ups is that you become capable of owning how your body rises from the ground and lowers itself to the ground in numerous ways with ease and control. Getting up from the ground shouldn't be a struggle. It should be graceful. And getting down to the ground shouldn't be a fall or collapse. It should be the ability to gracefully resist the force of gravity as well. This may not be the case for you at this moment, but it can be. You may need to surround yourself with objects that help you lower yourself down and pull yourself up.

---

[18]   http://www.usatoday.com/story/news/2015/02/26/sitting-rising-test-life-expectancy-fitness/24076407/.

If so, that is a great place to start. Remember, start where you are. It is okay if you need practice getting up and down from a bed before you dare get down on the floor. Once again, the bed is a wonderful place to start, as long as you start. With time and effort, you will get stronger and your ability to move will become more graceful. It will.

Don't be afraid of the floor or the ground. It is the one place you can always go, no matter where you are, to get stronger and move better.

16

IT'S TOO EASY NOT TO DO

"Engage."

—Captain Jean-Luc Picard on
Star Trek: The Next Generation

Now that we've looked at foundational movements and structural building movements, all we have to do now is get started. For some of us, experience has taught us that getting started is easier said than done, and for others, experience has taught us that getting started is one thing, but keeping that started thing going is another thing altogether.

The truth is, becoming strong doesn't have to be laborious, tedious, or torturous. It can be something you enjoy, especially as your newfound strength gives way to newfound freedoms. If you make it habit, becoming strong can also be sort of easy. Remember, the habit of strength is really designed to be our movement default. We were made to move, and we were made to be strong through the movements we make.

You didn't have a choice to be strong as a child. You simply became strong by moving through your default movement program. As an adult, you have to choose to be strong. This is really the starting point. Once you've made the choice to be strong, you have to engage—every single day.

You need to move to stay healthy. It's as simple as that. If you do not move, i.e. you sit in a chair all day, you will lose your health and your strength will deteriorate and you will become convinced that your body is betraying you.

Once you choose to be strong, you must act on your choice and start building your habit of strength. For the remainder of this book, I illustrate simple ways to establish movement habits, increase your strength, and become as strong as you want to be. These are just starting points and ideas to help you start where you are. One size won't fit all, but all will find a size that fits. Find what works for you and mold it to your lifestyle.

17

THE EASY HABITUAL
STRENGTH METHOD

If habits are built by simple addition, this beginner's routine is an attempt to start adding up some life-changing numbers. This routine is also an attempt to remove excuses. There is minimum equipment needed, if any, and the time commitment is less than twenty minutes per day. If you're a beginner and you're looking for a place to start, this is a good place for you:

Monday

1. Breathe ten consecutive diaphragmatic breaths
2. Nod your head up and down ten times
3. Roll back and forth ten times
4. Rock back and forth ten times
5. Perform ten marching cross-crawls
6. Perform ten minutes of get-ups

Get-ups:

Lie down on your back and stand up. Then lie back down on your back. Do this in as many different ways as you can for ten minutes. If you need props to help you get down to the floor and to help you get up from the floor, it's okay. Use what you need to use. Rest as you need to rest. When ten minutes has expired, you're done!

Monday night practice breathing with your diaphragm for five minutes. Keep your mouth closed, place your tongue on the roof of your mouth and breathe in and out through your nose.

Tuesday

1. Breathe ten consecutive diaphragmatic breaths
2. Nod your head up and down ten times
3. Roll back and forth ten times
4. Rock back and forth ten times
5. Perform ten marching cross-crawls
6. Baby crawl around your house for five minutes—Get some knee pads and crawl around while keeping your head held up, so you can see where you are going.
7. Next, *climb a mountain* (see below) with pushups and squats for ten minutes. Do what you can do, rest as you need to, climb as high as you can for ten minutes. Record how high you get so you can measure your improvement from week to week
8. Rock back and forth ten times.

How to climb a mountain:

Perform one pushup, then one squat. Then perform two pushups and two squats. Then three and three, four and four, and so on. Climb up to ten pushups and ten squats and then come back down, performing nine and nine, eight and eight, all the way back down to one and one.

If you were to climb all the way up to ten pushups and ten squats and then descended all the way back down to one pushup and one squat, you will have performed 100 pushups and 100 squats!

Climbing a mountain has its own built-in warm-up. It eases you in, you climb up high, the altitude gets thin, you get tired, then you climb down, and enjoy the built-in cool-down.

Tuesday night before bed practice slow head nods for five minutes.

Wednesday

1. Breathe ten consecutive diaphragmatic breaths
2. Nod your head up and down ten times
3. Roll back and forth ten times
4. Rock back and forth ten times
5. Perform ten marching cross-crawls
6. Perform *heavy* frontload carry (see below) for ten minutes—Do what you can, rest as you need to
7. Perform marching cross-crawls for three minutes.

What is a *heavy* frontload carry?

First of all, heavy is relative, but find a weight that challenges you. On a scale of one to ten, one being a feather, and ten being an elephant, find something in the six to seven range.

In a frontload carry, you are also going to practice hinging. Your task is to find a weight (dumbbell, kettlebell, sandbag, log, small child, or whatever), pick it up by folding at your hips (hinging) while you keep your chest proud (think Superman) and your gaze on the horizon. Then hold the weight out in front of you, chest high, and walk ten yards. Put it down the same way you picked it up. Turn around, pick it up again and walk back the same ten yards. Repeat this over and over again until your allotted time has expired.

Wednesday night before bed practice the modified windshield wiper for five minutes.

Thursday

1. Breathe ten consecutive diaphragmatic breaths
2. Nod your head up and down ten times
3. Roll back and forth ten times
4. Rock back and forth ten times
5. Perform ten marching cross-crawls
6. Perform ten minutes of get-ups
7. Perform walking single leg deadlifts (see below) for five minutes

Walking single leg deadlifts

Walking single leg deadlifts are a way to walk and hinge on one leg at a time. If you are standing on your left leg, you want to fold at your left hip while you reach back with your right leg, as if trying to touch the wall behind you. You are also going to simultaneously reach down towards the floor with your right hand. Then you unfold, or stand up, take a step forward with your right leg, hinge on the right leg, reach back with the left leg, and touch the floor with your left hand. Oh, also, keep your chest proud, like Superman, and hold your gaze on the horizon.

I know it sounds like a lot. These will challenge your balance and stability—and you're welcome. SLDLs also strengthen your low back, your butt, and the backs of your legs—again, you're welcome.

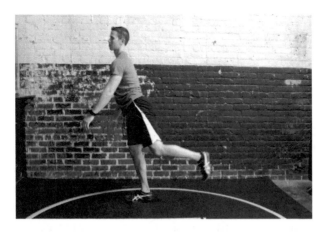

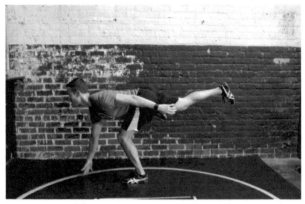

Seriously, If you get good at this movement, it'll change your life. Things like putting on socks and shoes while standing will become so easy.

Thursday night before bed practice rocking for five minutes.

Friday

1. Breathe ten consecutive diaphragmatic breaths
2. Nod your head up and down ten times
3. Roll back and forth ten times
4. Rock back and forth ten times
5. Perform ten marching cross-crawls

6. Perform Isometric Doorway pulls for six second pulls, for five minutes
7. Perform crawls to standing for ten minutes

Why isometric doorway pulls?

Well, pulls are the only major movement we haven't covered in the week. So we need to find a way to get them in our habitual routine. I don't know what resources you have available but I'm guessing you have a doorway. Remember, this is a routine for beginners, and it requires little to no equipment. Having said that, this routine can still benefit and strengthen the elite athlete. Finally, in case you are wondering, yes, isometric pulls can make you stronger.

To perform an isometric doorway pull, stand in front of an open doorway, brace yourself against the doorway with your top hand and push against the doorway then pull against the doorway with your bottom hand. Pull with 70 percent effort for six seconds and continue to breathe (with your diaphragm). What is 70 percent effort? It's that place where you are putting enough tension on the doorway to notice your muscles are really working. It's not everything you've got, but it's kind of close. Then, switch hands and repeat this over and over for five minutes. Rest as you need to and be sure not to hold your breath.

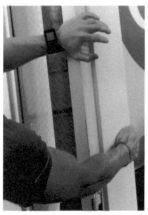 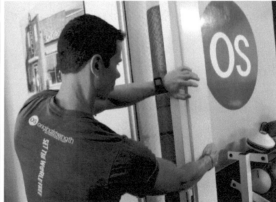

Crawling to stand

In this drill, we are simply crawling four to six steps and then standing up, and then getting back down to crawl. Repeat this over and over again for ten minutes. This can be done baby crawling on the hands and knees or by crawling on the hands and feet. If you choose to crawl on your hands and feet, remember to keep your head up and your butt down.

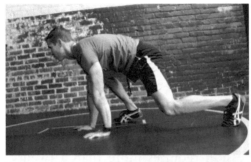

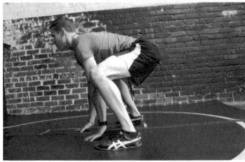

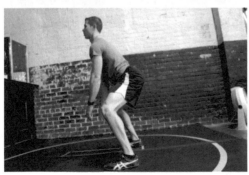

Friday night before bed practice breathing with and from your diaphragm for five minutes.

Saturday

1. Breathe ten consecutive diaphragmatic breaths
2. Nod your head up and down ten times
3. Roll back and forth ten times
4. Rock back and forth ten times
5. Perform ten marching cross-crawls
6. Go for a thirty to forty-five minute walk with purpose (see below)

Walk with purpose

Today, we are practicing carries with our own body. Walk with urgency, as if you have somewhere to go. Swing your arms from the shoulders and hold your gaze on the horizon. If you can, practice breathing through your nose while holding your mouth shut. Today's session requires more than a twenty-minute commitment, but this may be the most important movement session you've done all week.

If the weather is not cooperating, practice marching in doors for ten minutes. Again, swing your arms from the shoulders and land on the balls of your feet.

Saturday night before bed perform ten marching cross-crawls, rock back and forth ten times, perform ten rotations of the modified windshield wiper, nod your head up and down slowly ten times, and take ten deep, diaphragmatic breaths.

Sunday

1. Breathe ten consecutive diaphragmatic breaths
2. Nod your head up and down ten times
3. Roll back and forth ten times
4. Rock back and forth ten times

5. Perform ten marching cross-crawls
6. Do something fun today

Sunday night perform ten marching cross-crawls, rock back and forth ten times, perform ten rotations of the modified windshield wiper, nod your head up and down slowly ten times, and take ten deep, diaphragmatic breaths.

This routine is intended to help you establish a habit of movement and engagement while engraining good, efficient neural connections that also establish a foundation of reflexive strength, allowing your body to express the strength it was designed to have. If a person were to follow this plan for thirty days they could expect to move better, feel better, and be stronger.

After four weeks—if you enjoyed this routine and its results, you can easily progress the "work portions" (get-ups, "climbing mountains", marching, and SLDLs) by increasing the time by an additional five minutes. Remember, this is just a simple routine to get your habitual strength going strong. It won't be long until you're no longer a beginner. Sooner or later you will be looking to add more strength by progressing from this easy habitual strength method to a not-so-easy habitual strength method. Not-so-easy, but still simple. But, hey, that's a whole other book. The point is, this is a great place to start for building habitual strength, and it will take you a long, long ways because the numbers add up.

18

SIMPLE MATH

Let's look at how those numbers might add up to help you build the habit of strength. If you look at the thirty-day plan above, you might notice that every single day I had you perform at least ten marching cross-crawl touches. In thirty days, that will be at least 300 cross-crawl touches. In a year, that's 3,650 cross-crawl touches. On some of the days above, I had you do ten marching cross-crawl touches at night too. On Wednesdays I had you perform an extra three minutes of marching cross-crawl touches. If you did the above routine for a year, you'll be well over 10,000 marching cross-crawl touches in a year. Friends, that will literally pave the way for efficient neural connections that cannot be lost—it will pave the way for strength that will allow you to effortlessly move through life.

I understand your idea of strength may be a little more intense than simply performing cross-crawls. And while I could argue that the simple movement of cross-crawls could really grow into your idea of intense muscle building strength, let's play with the numbers in a way that may resonate with you a little better.

What if you did fifty pushups a day? Let's make this so simple you cannot *not* do it. What if you did ten pushups, five times a day, every day for a year? You could easily perform ten pushups, five times per day. You could easily do that every day of the year. That would be 18,250 pushups in a year. Again, that would not only lead to an efficient nervous system, but it would also lead to strong tendons and muscles that are ready for whatever life tries to throw at them. By the way, do you know if you performed ten pushups five times a day, every day of the year, you'll have also performed at least 1,825 get-ups? (You have to get down on the ground to perform pushups.) I wonder if that might help you develop the strength you need to live your life the way you want?

If you still think this method is too easy to work, look at it this way: You've already been applying this method your whole life, and it has gotten you the body you now have. Numbers add up. How many hours did you spend sitting in a chair yesterday? How about last week? How about last year? Let's assume the average person only spends six hours in a chair per day. That's about 2,190 hours spent sitting a year. Did you know that sitting for most of the day is detrimental to your health? How much do you think all those hours spent sitting, all those repetitions, add up when it comes to your health, or your lack of health?

You've already been playing simple math. You've already used numbers to build negative, or less-than-positive, habits. So why then, couldn't simple math—adding positive movements to your life—impact your health in a positive way? You just have to consistently add up the numbers and repetitions by making the right movements. The right movements aren't complicated. Your body is already preprogramed with them—so if you have reflexive strength, all the moves you make are the right moves.

19

Consistency and Living in the Middle

Rocky: "There's three of him out there."
Paulie: "Hit the one in the middle

—Sylvester Stallone, *Rocky IV*

There is a flow to everything, a way, or a path. Building habitual strength, strength made through your habits, is about finding that flow for your life. You cannot live in the land of extremes and expect to find the path that works for you. Do too little, live a sedentary life, and your body will decay, weaken, and become fragile. Do too much, try extreme means of fitness, or whatever, and your body will wear out, weaken, maybe get injured, and become fragile.

Unfortunately, when it comes to being healthy, many people live at the poles—in other words, they live in the extremes. Vitality is found in the middle. Listen, you can become as strong as you want to be and live the life you want to live by finding your flow and living in the middle. The key to this, the out-in-the-open secret is consistency. Consistency is the secret sauce that guides the path you should travel. Through consistent engagement, moving on purpose and moving often, you can become healthy and strong—without hurting yourself, without burning out, and without giving up.

There is no force more powerful than rushing, moving water. A raging river can effortlessly remove anything in its path. The amazing thing about raging rivers is they're comprised of individual drops of water. One drop at time, drops coming together, drops becoming trickles, trickles become streams, streams becoming rivers. That's how it's done. You can live your life in such a way that the individual actions you consistently take start to form neural pathways, much like individual molecules of water create a river. Consistent actions also form a body that becomes strong and capable. Much like how a raging river effortlessly removes obstacles in its path, you too will find that things that were once hard or difficult become easy. It becomes easy to move every day, it becomes easy to eat the right foods, it becomes easy to actually move heavy things and move the way "young" people move.

Live in the middle and find your flow. Once you accomplish this and fuel it with consistent engagement, strength is effortless and health is simply yours for as long as you want it. You don't have to participate in extreme ninety-day plans that are unsuitable for ninety-one days, or even twenty days for that matter. You don't have to run marathons. You don't need to spend two hours in the gym every day. You don't need to crawl out of an exercise class barely able to stand. All you have to do is consistently move with purpose every day. It can begin with the simple plan I outlined above. Think of the Easy Habitual Strength Method as three atoms—two hydrogen and one oxygen—that create drops of water that flow to create a stream of momentum that eventually turn into a river of strength.

20

SIMPLE RULES FOR NUTRITION

*"And the most important thing, the one thing you
must never forget: no matter how much he cries,
no matter how much he begs . . . never,
never feed him after midnight."*

—Randall Peltzer's character in *Gremlins*

Nutritionally, most of us don't live in the middle. One of the largest reasons people don't feel well, or have the body they want, is because our nutritional views and practices are out of balance. Handle your food intake the same way I've coached you to approach movement and exercise. That's right: Find your flow, and be consistent. Skip the extremes. Choose to consistently eat well. This means you don't need a spicy juice fast, and you don't have to go on extreme diets—or any diet. You simply need to consistently own your choices—this means making wise choices, which isn't always easy.

In America, nutrition has become tricky. We've created nutritional schisms, conspiracies, dogmas, and prisons. We've made food a villain and ourselves victims. It's all a giant mess. There's just too much noise when it comes to how we're supposed to eat. It's time to find a way to regain balance when it comes to our eating habits.

Let me say right now, I don't have all the answers when it comes to nutrition. I have my own beliefs about food, but I will not tell you they are gospel. Having said that, my principles about nutrition serve me well; they keep me grounded when I start to become aware of all the "nutritional" noise. I hope these principles help you find balance and give you guidance when the storms of nutrition begin to blow. As I discuss these principles, please know there are always exceptions, like allergies and preferences.

Principle #1: If God made it, it's probably okay to eat. Heck, it may even be good for you. If man made it, you should probably at least pause to consider if it is the right choice for your body and your desires.

I believe the closer your food is to its natural state, there is a good chance it's good for you. I'm not talking about cooking or not cooking your food. I'm talking about eating food that's from a farm, a field, a pasture, or an ocean. When food is highly processed, or it no longer resembles anything you could find in nature, then it's likely not all that good for you.

Principle #2: The longer the shelf-life of your food, the shorter your shelf-life. Foods commonly found in a supermarket are designed to last a long time. This affects profitability of both the manufacturer and the supermarket. It also affects your overall health, in a negative way. You probably don't need to eat a great deal of food preservatives to stay healthy, right? Foods found in nature, and by nature, are perishable and they really don't last long in the supermarket. Fresh, natural food has a short shelf-life, but it may increase your shelf-life. Simply put, Principle #2 echoes Principle #1.

Principle #3: It's your responsibility. How you eat and the choices you make about food are ultimately yours. Own them. You may not know all the ins and outs of nutrition, but you should have a pretty good intuition about what may be good for your body and what may not be good for your body. No one makes you eat anything you don't want to eat. Even if you don't know what foods are best for you to eat, you can learn. Educate yourself. Google is all the rage. But when in doubt, look to priciples 1 and 2 and own your choices.

Principle #4: Don't live in extremes. This is about living in the middle right? Let me help you. Fat is not evil. Don't avoid it, you can't live well without it. Carbs aren't the devil's plaything. You need carbs too. Also, cooking does denature protein. It's okay to cook your food.

Don't put your faith in a diet. Learn how to trust yourself. Living in the extremes with your approach to nutrition will set you up for frustration and failure.

21

RESPONSIBILITY

"With great power, comes great responsibility."

—Uncle Ben's character in *Spiderman*

Speaking of diets, here is the real deal about what you need to know when it comes to your nutrition. Diets don't work—at least not in the long run. Statistically speaking, that is. In fact, current statistics indicate that dieting is a consistent predictor of weight gain.[19]

If diets don't work, what does? Honesty and ownership. When it comes to eating well and being healthy, being honest with yourself and owning your decisions is the way to building healthy eating habits that will last you a lifetime. Know that your health is more important than your emotions, your boredom, or how you "feel." People eat when they are sad, they eat when they are mad, they eat when they are bored, they eat when they feel hungry, or they eat because they are on the couch. In all of these situations, none of them have anything to do with whether or

---

[19]   http://newsroom.ucla.edu/releases/Dieting-Does-Not-Work-UCLA-Researchers-7832.

not they actually need to eat. They all have to do with their state of mind or their lack of commitment to what they really want.

Be honest. You really do want to be healthy. You don't want to be obese. You don't want to have heart problems or diabetes. You don't want major health problems because you've eaten crap. No one does. But not everyone takes ownership of this desire to have good health. Instead, many people play victim to their circumstances, their emotions, or their excuses.

Eating healthy really doesn't have to be hard. It has to do with making decisions, deciding to eat natural foods, deciding to prepare your own meals versus eating at a fast-food restaurant, or deciding you're not going to eat simply because you're bored and you don't know what else to do. Do you need to eat candy? Do you need to eat cupcakes? Do you need to eat a twenty-ounce steak? Only you can honestly answer these questions. By the way, there is nothing wrong with eating these things as long as you own the decision. The key to eating well is taking responsibility for your actions and your choices.

You have to understand you have the awesome power of choice. The choices you make today, the consistent habitual choices you make, will reveal the body and the health you have chosen. In other words, you are responsible for what and how you eat. This means you are responsible for the outcome of your decisions. The state of your health today is due to the eating habits you've had prior to today. The state of your health in five years will be due to the eating habits you keep, create, and decide to have today. That's really good news, by the way. You can decide to have health and strength and then put action to your decision by creating habits through consistent thoughts, choices, and actions.

22

TIPS FOR EATING WELL

If you really don't know about food and how it affects your body, I encourage you to learn. Find books on nutrition, not diets, but nutrition. Search the Internet for sound information—don't fall for gimmicky ads about diets, weight loss, or cures. Search out solid information about nutrition, about how your body uses carbs, protein, and fats, and how and why you need vitamins and minerals to properly function. I'm a nutrition geek, so I've read a lot of nutrition books. One of my favorites is *Nourishing Traditions* by Sally Fallon. It talks about the history of food, how and why to prepare it, and why you need it.

What follows are some tips I think may help you in your quest to become strong and healthy through your nutritional habits:

- When you go grocery shopping, stay on the outside edges of the store. Most grocery stores are set up so that the natural foods are found along the outside of the store and the processed foods are found towards the middle. Fruits, vegetables, meats, eggs, and dairy can all be found along the outside of most grocery stores. Foods that come in boxes with cartoon characters can be found in the middle of the stores. If it's found along the outside, it's probably good for you. If it's found towards the inside and in a box, it's probably heavily processed and designed to last a great deal of time on the store shelf. This means you don't need it.

- When you're buying your fruits and vegetables, buy brightly colored ones. Deep reds, purples, and greens usually pack more nutritional value.

- If you don't buy junk food in the store, it will be hard for you to eat it in your home.

- Keep a food journal! Record what you eat, how much you eat, and when you eat it. Be honest when you do this. A food journal provides you a good snapshot of your daily eating habits. And it is a way to help keep yourself accountable.

- Prepare your meals at night for the next day at work. Take your meals to work. Go prepared. If you arrive at work with your meal in hand, you don't have to be a victim of the circumstances that your workday throws at you. A great tasting, healthy sandwich carried to work can spare you from the double cheeseburger you might buy at a fast-food restaurant.

- Tell your friends you are wanting and trying to eat healthy. If you let your friends know, they may respect your decision and even support you. If they don't, at least you verbalized your desire, which puts it out in the open making it more real to you. This tip also works for beginning new exercise programs. If you tell others, you may find support or even a companion who wants to embark on the journey with you. There really can be strength in numbers. If, however, your friends ridicule you, belittle you, or try to sabotage you, go ahead and remove them from your inner circle.

- This last tip is from client experience. You should know that a gram of alcohol has about 7.2 calories in it. It has almost twice the caloric value of a gram of sugar, and it is burned like a simple sugar. I'm not saying you shouldn't enjoy a spirited beverage every now and then. I'm simply saying numbers add up. If you like to have a six-pack every Saturday, consider a "lite" six-pack, or consider enjoying four beers instead of six, one glass of wine instead of four. Incidentally, if you do decide to keep a food journal, alcohol gets written down too!

- Life happens. If you absolutely have to go to a fast-food restaurant, don't get the fries. Don't get the soft drink. Don't get the milkshake. Use your judgment. Your honest judgment.

- Understand that being strong and healthy has a great deal to do with how you move and how often you move. But, being healthy and having a healthy body weight, composition, and physique is more dependent on what you eat.

23

FIND YOUR FLOW

"The only rules that really matter are these: what a man can do and what a man can't do."

—Captain Jack Sparrow in *Pirates of the Caribbean*

Can you put together enough "drops of change" to create the river of strength you want to have in your body? In your life? The choice is yours. You can absolutely be as strong as you want to be and live the life you want to live. You can overcome bad habits and you can create new, more desirable habits.

You have a brain and a body that are designed for routine. You get to create the routine that determines what you can achieve mentally and physically.

The ideas, movements, and routines in this book really can set you on your way to building habitual strength, strength that is yours because of the habits you keep through the choices you make. You are completely capable of becoming healthier and improving your life, one movement at a time.

The methods outlined in this book need not only be applied towards exercise. If there is an area of your life that you want to improve, or an area of your life where you want to create new habits, you can apply the same method of simple addition. What would happen if every day, you told your spouse how much you loved them? Or, what if you did something nice for them every day? Do you think you could create a simple habit that might dramatically improve your relationship? What if you want to improve your relationship with your kids? What if you spent just ten extra minutes with them each day? Maybe you play toss or tag with them. Maybe you just talk. What would that do for your children, and how would it impact the rest of their lives? I mention this because these too are habits—habits we create through simple addition. It's a similar, but different sort of habitual strength, yes?

We are all capable of change. We're all capable of almost anything. If you want to absolutely improve your current condition, you can absolutely do it. You don't have to settle for bad health, weak relationships, or even a messy house. You can change. You can improve your life, your health, and your strength. A better life that reflects the healthy habits you create is waiting for you. It will take time and energy, but it's worth the effort. You're worth the effort!

LEARN MORE ABOUT ORIGINAL STRENGTH

Our mission is to change the world through movement. As the foundation for all movement for any activity, we teach health and fitness professionals a system that allows for improved patient and client results. We invite you to visit our website at OriginalStrength.net for more information. While on the site, please look at our workshops, videos (Movement Snax™), DVDs, equipment and other books. We want to help you move the way you were designed to.

To locate a coach in your area go to:
https://originalstrength.net/find-a-certified-coach

We have OS Certified Coaches located around the world.

www.originalstrength.net

"I am fearfully and wonderfully made."

—Psalm 139:14